An Addiction of Damaging Hair

Dennise Zepeda

Cover Design: Youth Vision Inc.
Editor: Mrs. Murphy (Teacher)
Copyrights © 2012 – Youth Vision Inc.
All rights reserved
Printed in the United States of America
www.youthvisioninc.org

Introduction

This book is about me (Dennise Zepeda) dying my hair and doing all sorts of things with it. Also, regarding my mother (Jennifer Zepeda) and my sister (Deana Zepeda). My mother is the one who is in charge and the one who gets me in trouble also punishes me (gives me consequences). My sister on the other hand, is my partner. The one who is like my partner in crime. The one who has my back all the time, no matter what. This book is like a diary.

Table Of Content

About The Author

My name is Dennise Zepeda. I wrote this
book basically about my hair and yeah.
I am 12 years old and in middle school. I go to
Bancroft Middle School.
I'm always coloring my hair so I decided to
write a book on my hair life.
My sister and my mom are involved in this
story, because (1) my sister helped me with my
hair; (2) my mom is the one that gives me
permission and it gets me in trouble if I don't
have permission and yeah. So I hope you
enjoyed the book.

Dennise Zepeda

CHAPTER 1

The Day My Mom Said No
>;/

Once me and my sister wanted to dye our hair. My hair was blonde and hers was black.

My mother replied, "No, you cannot dye your hair."

My sister and I begged her, "Please mom, we'll do anything you want us to do. We'll clean the whole entire house. ANYTHING!" She still said no. Then we stopped asking 'til one month passed by. I asked my mother again, "Mom can I dye my hair?" She replied, "No."

I was thinking to myself, "How can I convince her?" So I went on Facebook (a website for friends and family) , and put a status/ post saying, "How do you convince a mom to let you dye your hair?" Then my friend that goes to Madison Middle School (Priscilla) said, "Tell your mom you'll clean the whole house." Then I replied, "I already told her that, and she said no." Priscilla said, "Just clean the whole house without saying anything; be nice; be respectful.

Then ask her, and if she says no, don't whine. It won't help. Just keep trying. Eventually she will let you.

CHAPTER 2

The Day I Dyed My Hair ;D

I did so. Then I asked my mom, "Can I dye my hair? It's temporary dye. It comes off every time you take a shower." She said, "Yes, only if you vacuum and wash dishes." Then I said, "Okay, I'll do it." Then I did. A few days later I asked my sister, "Can you help me dye my hair?" She said, "Sure, why not?" Then I was like, "AW YEH." Another few days later I said to my sister , "Are you still gonna help me?" She said, "Yes, tonight we'll do your hair." Later that day (it was night time already) she said to me, "Are you ready?" and I said, "Yes." She interrupted me saying, "You know you have to bleach your hair right?" Then I said, "No?" as if I wasn't sure. Then my sister said, "Well, you have to in order for the color to come out nice and bright," Then I said, "Is mom going to be okay with it?" My sister replied, "No." In my mind I was saying to myself, "What would happen?. . .

I really want this. I've been wanting this for a while and this is my only chance to do it. I already bought the TEMPORARY dye." Then I said to my sister, "Go for it. Mom won't know." She said, "Are you sure?" Then I said, "Yes, I'm sure." So she went for it. She applied it with an applicator brush. It's a brush with a tail at the end to help part hair into pieces sections. She did it very neat. It took almost an hour or more! When she was done, she put foil paper on the pieces that she bleached so my hair would turn lighter faster. We left the bleach on for about 24 minutes. If we left the bleach on for too long my hair would literally fall off, since there is so much chemicals in the bleach. Then I washed it out and my hair was like a whitish blonde. My hair was literally fried because of the chemicals.

CHAPTER 3

When I Washed Out The TEMPORARY Dye

^___<3

I waited two days to insert the pink TEMPORARY dye. I waited two days because I didn't want to damage my hair. The day after I bleached it, my hair was an orangey blondish color. It was better than the whitish blonde. That day I went to the movies with my sister, her boyfriend, and her boyfriend's older brother. They were saying I looked so different, that I didn't look twelve years old, that I looked more like a teenager in their early fifteens. They didn't like the hair color.

My sister's boyfriend's mother took us home. When we got home, a few minutes later my mother called saying, "What are you guys doing?" We said back to her, "Nothing much just here. We went to the movies." My mom said, "Oh okay, anything new?" Then I said, "My hair is sorta blondish." Then she stayed quiet. When she was about to say something I interrupted her saying, "I'm putting in pink so it doesn't look bad." Then she hung up.

Later that day I put in the pink TEMPORARY dye. I waited about 15 minutes until it got hard. It was time to wash it out. When I had gotten out of the shower, my hair was as pink as a pink valentine card! I was almost freaking out even though I liked it. Then my mother called saying, "The pink is temporary right?"
"Yes," I replied.

She asked, "How long does it take for the dye to wash out?"

I said, "Three months."

Then my mom started freaking out saying she didn't give me permission when she did.

She said on the phone, "When I get home I'm going to dye your hair dark brown."

I said, "Okay."

I only did my bangs and the bottom of my hair.

When my mother got home, she had the brown dye. Then she started dying my hair. When I got out of the shower from washing the dye out, it looked dark. When it started to dry, it looked reddish. I was starting not to like it. Then days later my hair was turning a light brown. It looked nice but since I was going to a new school, Bancroft Middle School, I had to dye it black. I don't know why but my mother said I have to find a way to dye it black. So I found away. I bought my own black dye and dyed my hair myself with no help at all.

CHAPTER 4

When My Hair Was Black
c:

My hair was pitch black. When I was dying it, my gloves looked purple, as if I was dying my hair purple! I hate the color purple so it was like a nightmare. So I bought a blacker hair dye, volume 20, so it can be really black. The dye was still purple, sadly.

I left the black dye in for about 35 minutes. It was burning a lot and it itched. After 35 minutes, I washed the dye out. It was kind of still stinging when I was washing it. I couldn't use shampoo or the conditioner. I had to use this conditioner that came with the black hair dye. I had two of those conditioners.

I had to use that kind of conditioner that came with the dye so my hair won't get damaged a lot, and so that when I'm done washing it, my hair is soft and shiny.

I had to use that conditioner for like about three weeks, for longer lasting black hair. If i didn't use that conditioner, my hair would be all damaged , and the color would just be dull.

My hair was really soft and shiny when i finished washing out the dye. When it dried i straightened it for the next day. The next day was school.

CHAPTER 5

When I Bleached My Hair Again
^___^

A few weeks later, I got tired of the color

So I bleached my bangs, so that they would turn out to a lighter color. And I didn't ask my mom. When my mother got home, she was like totally freaking out about my hair.

I was telling her,

"It's just hair! It'll grow out."

My mom was like, "It doesn't matter. You're supposed to ask for permission, not just go off and do whatever you want."

I stayed quiet.
Then she said, "Do you know the damage that you're doing to your hair? You're killing your hair. You're frying it; you are damaging it so much."

I didn't say anything because I knew she was right.

My mom let me keep the blonde for a while. Then she made me dye it black. I bought my own dye..... AGAIN. It was manic panic hair dye, the most awesome hair dye in the world. Says me.

I have a lot of arguments with my mom about. . .

My hair. She keeps telling me that I'm damaging it. I know I am. She doesn't have to tell me.
After a little while she got over it. Everything was back to normal (almost).

CHAPTER 6

My Sister Dyed Her Hair. . . Without Permission
;o

So one day my sister said to me,

"Heeeeey, I'm going to dye my hair."

Then I said, "Oh, what color?" She said, "Red, like a neon red."

I said to her, "Did you ask mom?"

She said, "Nahh, she doesn't have to know."

I told her, "You know mom's going to get mad if you don't tell her?" She said,

"You dyed your hair without permission and she didn't do anything but tell you things and lecture you," I said.

"Really. That doesn't mean she'll do the same to you."

There was an awkward silence.

My sister wanted me to buy the dye for her, the one that I used for my hair (Manic Panic) I told her, "Nah, you can get it yourself. If I can, you can."

She said to me, "Whatever. I'll Do It MySelf." I was fine with it. She went to the mall and got herself some hair dye. Then at night she dyed her hair with my help ^_^. It was a really bright color, like a tomato.

Eventually my mom found out. My sister got in more trouble than I did. She got her cell phone, laptop, and her T.V taken.

Haha! I was laughing so hard. I told her that she should have asked, and since she was older, my mom would have said yes.

I should've told my sister that. Anyway I dyed my hair purple, and yes I asked my mom, and she said, "Yes."

I dyed the blonde part purple because me and my friend were making a bet on who can pull an all nighter (an all nighter is when you don't sleep at all) and apparently I lost.

As you can see, the bet was to dye your hair purple if you lost.

We both hated the color purple, so that's why we betted.

CHAPTER 7

Me and My Sister Dye Our Hair

xD

Ah, the story of my life. Me and my sister dyed our hair black. . . again.

We had permission this time because our mom didn't like our random hair color.

My sister and I dyed our hair with each other at the same time. It was really cool because we were talking about stuff we like. It was a good day.

It was kind of weird when me and my sister saw each other with black hair because we were like, "Omg! (Oh my gosh) we look the same."

Then I said, "Err not really, just our hair." She was like, "Hmm. . . We are twins now!"

Then I walked away. It got awkward.

CHAPTER 8

Me Going to a New School

;/

Aha, so, I'm at a new school called Bancroft Middle School.

It's a really cool school, but since my hair is black, people have been asking me if I'm goth or emo. It bugs me; it's annoying.

Just because I have a certain style to my hair does not mean I'm "emo."

This kid went up to me and said, "Hey, are you emo?"

Which was like the first thing he said to me not even,

"What's your name?" or "What school do you come from?"

Like really. Who says that to a new person in the school?

I just ignored it and said, "No I am not." Then I walked away.

Luckily I know a lot of people but hang out with a little bit of people ._.

Everyone is calling my name:
"Hey, Dennise."

Calling me: "The new girl." It's pretty cool. I feel noticed.

So yeah the school is fun. I like how some girls have their own sense of style.

CHAPTER 9

My Mom Won't Let Me Straighten My Hair
D;

So like about the first week of school, my mom let me straighten my hair.

Then when I started getting use to the school, my mom wouldn't let me straighten my hair. When my mom picked me up after school she said,

"I don't want you straightening your hair anymore."

Then I asked, "Why?"

She said, "Because one, you look like a boy. Two , you're damaging your hair. Three, you just dyed your hair so that's even more damage."

I said to her, "Well, I like my hair. It's my sense of style."

My mom said to me, "You can't straighten your hair." Then I said, "Well, what about what I want?" She didn't reply.

I wanted to straighten my hair so bad that I kept bugging; my mom and asking her if I can. Then she got mad and said,

"Do whatever you want to do."

When she said that, I didn't want to anymore. I still did but if I would have done it, she would have gotten mad, so I didn't. She might forget by next week. I might do my hair (straighten it) by then.

So my school is turning out to be an okay school.

I meet new people almost every day and every single friend I make, says they like my hair. I miss my old school.

Things happen for a reason.

The next color I'm going to dye my hair is blue.

Yes, I'm going to dye all of my hair.

CHAPTER 10

My Best Friend
<3

So, I notice I say so a lot. Anyway I have I new, best friend. His name is Honorato. Anyway, he's really nice, and funny.

We have lots in common. We like the same music, colors, and stuff. So yeah, we have the same hair style. He's kind of like a boy version of me, and I'm like a girl version of him.He says he used to have hair slicked forward, but I can't see it. His hair is kind of like mine, but a little bit of a shorter version.

Anyway, my new school is small. My other school was way bigger than this one. This school has floors, 3 floors. I'm not used to floors >.<. I'm used to like flat schools. I really miss my old school. So yeah, Honorato picks me up from my bus stop and we hang out. He's really cool. At my other school, we used to hang out a lot after school.

We would go to the ice cream truck, the mall, Rite Aid, El Pollo Loco, and Starbucks. After that we would walk around the school a few times, then wait for our parents to pick us up.

It's not the same over here. The classes are too long >.<, oh well.

My friends are really cool, and nice to me ^___^. Some are funny, but yeah, what sucks is that this school has a free dress day like about every six months.

I could wait. I hope this school year goes well.

Names Of Characters

Mom: Jennifer Zepeda <3

Sister: Deana Zepeda<3

Me: Dennise Zepeda <3

New Best friend: Honortato DeGuzman <3

Dedication

I would like to dedicate this book to my best friend Summer Hoskins, and my sister Deana Zepeda, because Summer is the one who was with me when I got everything, She bleached her hair with me.
Deana was the who helped me with my hair all the time, and I was the one who help her with her hair. So, yeah.

HAIR TIPS

HAIR TIPS

HAIR TIPS

HAIR TIPS